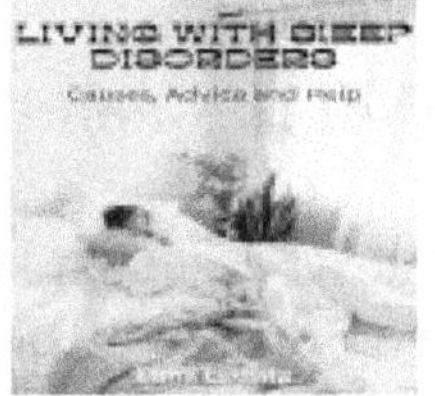
LIVING WITH SLEEP
DISORDERS
Causes, Advice and Help

Introduction to sleep problems

Sleep problems affect many people and can manifest themselves in different ways. Some people have difficulty falling asleep, while others have difficulty staying asleep or waking up early. Sleep problems can lead to various health problems, such as fatigue, mood swings and concentration problems. It is important to take sleep problems seriously and look for solutions to improve health and well-being. Sleep is an important part of human life and has many functions. During sleep, the body regenerates, the brain processes information and the metabolism is regulated. Sufficient and restful sleep is necessary to lead a healthy life. There are many reasons for sleep problems. One of the most common reasons is stress. Stress can make it difficult to fall asleep or cause you to wake up at night and not be able to relax again. Other reasons can be anxiety, depression, pain, irregular bedtimes and certain medications. Sleep disorders such as sleep apnea or restless legs syndrome can also lead to sleep problems. If you have sleep problems, there are many things you can do to improve your sleep quality. One way is to optimize your sleeping environment. Make sure your bedroom is cool, dark and quiet. Also, avoid stimulants such as caffeine or alcohol before bedtime as they can disrupt sleep. Another way to improve your sleep quality is to introduce a regular bedtime routine. Try to go to bed and get up at the same time every day, even on weekends. A regular bedtime will help your body prepare for sleep and regulate the natural sleep cycle. Relaxation techniques such as yoga or progressive muscle relaxation can also help to calm the body and mind and improve sleep. A healthy diet and sufficient exercise can also help to improve the quality of sleep. In some cases, sleep problems can be more serious and require medical treatment. If your sleep problems persist or worsen, you should see a doctor. A doctor can diagnose sleep disorders and recommend appropriate treatment options. There are also various medications and therapies that can help treat sleep disorders. However, sleeping pills should only be taken as directed by a doctor and only for a limited period of time, as they can be addictive and lead to other health problems.

What are sleep disorders?

Sleep disorders are a widespread phenomenon and refer to a disruption of normal sleep patterns. There are many different types of sleep disorders, some of which can be very serious and can have a significant impact on a person's health and well-being. A sleep disorder can be caused by a variety of factors, including psychological, medical and environmental factors. The most common causes of sleep disorders include stress, anxiety, depression, pain, respiratory system disorders such as sleep apnea and insomnia. Sleep disorders can have many different symptoms, including difficulty falling asleep or staying asleep, nightmares, nighttime awakenings, restless sleep, daytime sleepiness, difficulty concentrating, irritability and fatigue. These symptoms can vary in severity depending on the type of sleep disorder. Insomnia is one of the most common sleep disorders. It occurs when a person has difficulty falling asleep or staying asleep. This can be caused by a variety of factors, such as stress, anxiety, depression, pain or irregular sleep patterns. Insomnia can cause a person to feel tired and listless during the day, have difficulty concentrating and their mood may be affected. Another common sleep disorder is sleep apnea. This occurs when breathing is disturbed during sleep and the person wakes up several times a night to catch their breath. This can lead to impaired sleep quality and fatigue during the day. People with sleep apnea also have an increased risk of cardiovascular disease and other health problems. Narcolepsy is another sleep disorder characterized by sudden and uncontrolled sleep attacks. These can occur at any time of the day and can force a person to fall asleep during the day, even if they are in an active or dangerous situation. People with narcolepsy may also have symptoms such as cataplexy, hallucinations and sleep paralysis. There are also a variety of environmental factors that can contribute to sleep disturbances, such as noise, light, temperature and sleep environment. For example, noise from the street or neighbors can make it difficult to fall asleep or interrupt sleeping through the night. A bedroom that is too bright can inhibit the production of melatonin, a hormone responsible for the sleep-wake cycle.

The importance of sleep

Sleep is a vital function of the human body and plays an important role in maintaining physical and mental health. Although everyone has different sleep needs, everyone needs sufficient sleep to function optimally. In this article, we will explore the importance of sleep and the effects of sleep deprivation on the body and mind. Sleep is a process in which the body and mind rest and renew themselves. During sleep, the body goes through different stages characterized by different brain activities and body functions. A typical sleep cycle consists of five different stages, each lasting between 90 minutes and two hours. During sleep, the body goes through these stages several times in order to recover and regenerate. The importance of sleep is manifold. Adequate sleep is important for physical health, as the body carries out important repair and maintenance work during sleep. Lack of sleep can lead to a variety of health problems, including diabetes, cardiovascular disease and obesity. Adequate sleep is also important for mental health. During sleep, the brain can consolidate memories, solve problems and develop creative ideas. However, a lack of sleep can have serious effects on the body and mind. Short-term sleep deprivation can lead to fatigue, irritability and concentration problems. Long-term sleep deprivation can lead to chronic fatigue, depression, anxiety and even hallucinations. Lack of sleep can also affect the immune system and increase the risk of infections. The effects of sleep deprivation on the body are numerous. Lack of sleep can alter the metabolism and lead to weight gain and obesity. Lack of sleep can also lead to an increase in blood pressure and cholesterol levels, which increases the risk of cardiovascular disease. Lack of sleep can also increase the risk of diabetes as it raises blood sugar levels and reduces insulin sensitivity. Lack of sleep can also lead to mental problems. It can affect mood and lead to depression and anxiety. Lack of sleep can also impair cognitive function and lead to memory problems and poor concentration. Chronic sleep deprivation can even damage the brain and lead to long-term effects. To understand the importance of sleep, it is important to understand the different stages of sleep.

Stages of sleep

The human body needs sleep to recover and regenerate. During sleep, the body goes through different stages, known as sleep stages. In total, there are four main stages of sleep, each characterized by distinctive brain activity and body reactions. The first stage of sleep is the falling asleep stage, also known as stage 1. In this stage, brain waves are slow and irregular. The body gradually relaxes and breathing and heartbeat slow down. This stage usually lasts only a few minutes. The second stage of sleep is stage 2, where brain waves become slower but periodic brain activity (spindles) also occur. Eye movements stop and muscle activity is reduced. A person spends most of their sleep in this stage. The third and fourth stages of sleep are also known as the deep sleep stages. Brain waves are slowest and most regular in these stages. Breathing and heartbeat are very slow and muscle activity is greatly reduced. Deep sleep is when the body regenerates the most. Hormone production also takes place at this stage. During deep sleep, it is difficult to interrupt sleep as the body is in a state of deep relaxation. If you are woken up at this stage, you often feel confused or disoriented. The body usually needs some time to wake up from this stage. The fourth stage of sleep is also known as "delta sleep", as the brain predominantly produces delta waves in this stage. These waves are very slow and deep. The delta sleep stage is usually the longest sleep stage that is passed during a night. During sleep, the body also goes through a phase known as REM (Rapid Eye Movement) sleep. This is the phase in which most dreams occur. During REM sleep, the brain waves are active and similar to those during wakefulness. The eyes move rapidly back and forth, and breathing and heartbeat become irregular. In REM sleep, the body is normally paralyzed to prevent the movements experienced in dreams from being carried out in waking life. During REM sleep, memory consolidation also takes place as the brain transfers information from short-term memory to long-term memory. REM sleep usually occurs about 90 minutes after falling asleep and lasts about 20-25% of the total sleep time.

Normal sleep

Normal sleep is a fundamental biological process that is essential for physical and mental health and well-being. It is a state of rest in which the body can regenerate and recover while the brain performs various tasks that are important for cognitive and emotional function. In this article, we will take a closer look at what normal sleep is, what phases it has and how much sleep we need. Sleep phases Sleep consists of different phases that vary in intensity and activity. Sleep stages are usually divided into two main categories: non-REM sleep and REM sleep. Non-REM sleep consists of three stages that differ in terms of brain activity and muscle tension. In the first stage of non-REM sleep, the body relaxes, breathing slows down and the heart rate decreases. Muscle tension decreases and eye movements slow down. Brain activity also decreases and hypnagogic hallucinations may occur, often described as sudden jerks or brief images. The second stage of non-REM sleep is deeper than the first stage. In this stage, muscle tension is further reduced and the brain begins to show slow wave activity. However, the body remains receptive to external stimuli, such as sounds. In the third stage of non-REM sleep, the deepest sleep occurs. In this stage, brain wave activity is at its slowest and muscle tension is at its lowest. The body is less receptive to external stimuli at this stage and it is more difficult to wake up. REM sleep, also known as dream sleep, is the fourth stage of sleep. In this stage, brain activity is very high and the eyes move quickly. The muscles are relaxed, but not as much as in the previous stages. REM sleep is important for learning and memory, as the brain processes and stores information during this stage. Normal sleep cycle A normal sleep cycle lasts around 90 to 110 minutes and consists of a sequence of non-REM and REM phases. The cycle begins with non-REM sleep and then moves on to REM sleep. A healthy adult goes through about four to six such cycles per night. How much sleep do you need? Sleep requirements vary from person to person and also depend on age. Newborns and infants need an average of 14 to 17 hours of sleep per day, while children aged 1 to 2 years should sleep around 11 to 14 hours. School-age children (6-13 years) need around 9 to 11 hours.

Causes of sleep disorders

Sleep disorders can have many causes and are a common problem affecting millions of people worldwide. This article discusses the main causes of sleep disorders. Stress and anxiety Stress and anxiety are common triggers of sleep disorders. When a person is stressed or anxious, their body can go into a state of heightened alert, making it harder to fall asleep and stay asleep. A stressed mind can also cause a person to constantly think and worry about their problems instead of relaxing and calming down. Depression Depression can also cause sleep disorders. People who suffer from depression may have difficulty falling asleep or staying asleep and may also feel very tired and exhausted during the day. Shift work People who work shifts are often prone to sleep disorders. When the body has to adapt to unfamiliar working hours, it can be difficult to regulate sleep patterns and get enough sleep. Jet lag Jet lag is a disruption of the sleep-wake cycle caused by traveling across multiple time zones. It can take a few days for the body to adjust to the new time zone, which can lead to sleep disturbances. Caffeine and alcohol Caffeine and alcohol can both cause sleep disturbances. Caffeine is a stimulant that keeps the body awake and can impair the ability to fall asleep. Alcohol can affect the quality of sleep and cause a person to wake up more frequently during the night. Medications Some medications can cause sleep disturbances, including certain antidepressants, blood pressure medications and steroids. If a person suspects that their medication is affecting their sleep quality, they should speak to their doctor to see if there are alternative medications that do not cause sleep disturbances. Sleep apnea Sleep apnea is a sleep disorder caused by cessation of breathing during sleep. It can lead to frequent awakenings during the night and poor sleep quality. If a person suspects that they are suffering from sleep apnea, they should see a doctor to get a diagnosis and appropriate treatment. Restless legs syndrome (RLS) Restless legs syndrome is a disorder caused by uncomfortable sensations in the legs that can cause a person to constantly move their legs in order to feel relief.

The role of lifestyle in sleep disorders

Insomnia is a common problem that affects many people. There are many different factors that can contribute to people having trouble falling asleep or staying asleep. One of the most important factors is lifestyle. A healthy lifestyle can help prevent or improve sleep disorders, while an unhealthy lifestyle can increase the risk of sleep disorders. In this article, we will take a closer look at the role of lifestyle in sleep disorders. Sleep is an important part of a healthy lifestyle. When we get enough sleep, we can concentrate better, improve our mood and improve our physical health. However, people who don't get enough sleep can experience a variety of problems, including cognitive impairment, mood problems and increased risk of diseases such as diabetes and heart disease. An unhealthy lifestyle can contribute to sleep disorders. One important factor is diet. A poor diet rich in sugary and fatty foods can make you feel energized but experience a decrease in energy levels later in the day, which can make it difficult to fall asleep. However, if you eat a balanced diet with plenty of vegetables, fruit, whole grains and lean protein, you can help ensure that your body has the energy it needs to move during the day and that it can relax and sleep at night. Exercise is another important part of a healthy lifestyle and can also help prevent sleep disorders. Regular exercise can help reduce stress and improve mood, which can help you sleep better. However, it's important to be mindful of when you exercise. Exercising just before bedtime can make you feel winded and make it difficult to fall asleep. It is recommended to stop exercising at least 2-3 hours before bedtime. Another important factor in sleep disorders is the consumption of stimulating substances such as caffeine and alcohol. Caffeine, which is found in coffee, tea and many carbonated drinks, can make you feel energized and keep you awake if you consume it just before bedtime. Alcohol can also make you feel relaxed and fall asleep faster, but it can also cause you to wake up more often during the night and sleep more restlessly. It is important to pay attention to your consumption of stimulants and reduce or avoid them if necessary to achieve good quality sleep.

The role of nutrition in sleep disorders

Sleep disorders are a widespread problem in today's society. There are many reasons why people have trouble falling asleep or staying asleep, but one often overlooked cause is diet. In this article, we will explore the role of diet in sleep disorders and how to promote a healthy diet to encourage a good night's sleep. A balanced diet is crucial for a good night's sleep. An unhealthy diet can lead to an imbalance of nutrients and hormones in the body, which can affect sleep. A diet high in refined sugar and carbohydrates but low in fiber and protein can destabilize blood sugar levels and lead to sleep disturbances. One way to promote a healthy diet is by including adequate fiber in the diet. Fiber is important for regulating blood sugar levels and helps protect the body from the negative effects of blood sugar fluctuations. Fiber-rich foods such as whole grains, vegetables and legumes can help keep blood sugar levels stable and improve sleep. Another way to promote a healthy diet is by eating enough protein. Protein is important for building and repairing tissues in the body, including the muscles and brain. A balanced diet should contain sufficient protein to support bodily functions. Protein-rich foods such as meat, fish, eggs and dairy products can help provide the body with the necessary nutrients to promote a good night's sleep. There are also certain foods that can help promote sleep. One example of this is tryptophan, an amino acid that is converted in the body into the hormone serotonin, which is responsible for regulating sleep and mood. Tryptophan-rich foods such as milk, chicken, cheese and nuts can help to supply the body with this important nutrient and improve sleep. Another example is foods that contain magnesium. Magnesium is an important mineral that is necessary for muscle relaxation and nervous system regulation. Magnesium-rich foods such as nuts, legumes and whole grains can help to supply the body with this important mineral and improve sleep. However, there are also certain foods and drinks that should be avoided to promote a good night's sleep. One example of this is caffeine, which is found in many drinks such as coffee, tea and energy drinks.

The role of stress in sleep disorders

Stress and sleep disorders are closely linked. Stress is a natural part of life and can even be helpful in certain situations. However, when stress becomes chronic, it can affect health and lead to a variety of physical and psychological problems, including sleep disorders. Sleep disorders can manifest themselves in a variety of ways, such as difficulty falling asleep or staying asleep, restless sleep or early morning awakenings. There are a variety of factors that can contribute to sleep disorders, but stress is one of the most common triggers. When we are stressed, our bodies produce stress hormones such as adrenaline and cortisol. These hormones help us react to a potential threat by speeding up our heartbeat, accelerating our breathing and tensing our muscles. However, this "fight or flight" mode is not only active during acute threats, but also during chronic stress, which is often caused by work, family or financial problems. When we are in a constant state of alert, this can disrupt our sleep cycle. Cortisol is normally produced in the morning and helps us to wake up and start the day. As the day progresses, cortisol production decreases, making way for the sleep hormone melatonin, which helps us fall asleep. However, when we are stressed, our cortisol production can remain high at night, keeping us awake and disrupting our sleep cycle. Stress can also lead to physical ailments that interfere with sleep. When we are stressed, our muscles tense up, which can lead to pain and tension. This can lead to restless sleep and sleep disorders. In addition, stress can also lead to gastroesophageal reflux, which can make it difficult to fall asleep. Another factor that links stress and sleep disorders is anxiety. When we are stressed, we tend to worry and be anxious. This anxiety can disrupt sleep and prevent us from falling asleep or sleeping through the night. In addition, the anxiety of sleep disturbance itself can lead to a vicious cycle where the anxiety of not being able to sleep leads to even more stress and sleep disturbance. There is also an interaction between sleep disorders and stress. Sleep disorders can cause us to feel stressed and overtired, which can increase stress and lead to a further increase in sleep disorders. This vicious cycle can be difficult to break and often requires comprehensive treatment. There are several ways to treat stress and sleep disorders.

Sleep disorders in children

Sleep disorders can occur in children of any age. From difficulty falling asleep to waking up frequently during the night or waking up too early in the morning, there are a variety of sleep problems that can occur in children. These sleep disorders can have a variety of causes, including stress, anxiety, poor sleeping habits or physical ailments. In this article, we will discuss some of the most common sleep disorders in children and provide tips on how to overcome these problems. One of the most common sleep disorders in children is insomnia. Children with insomnia have difficulty falling asleep and can lie awake in bed for hours. This sleep disorder can be caused by a variety of factors, including anxiety, stress, pain or an irregular sleep schedule. To help children with insomnia, it is important to establish a regular bedtime and reduce stress through relaxation exercises or calming techniques. It can also be helpful to reduce the use of electronic devices such as cell phones and tablets before bedtime. Another sleep disorder that can occur in children is night waking. Children who wake up frequently during the night may have difficulty falling back asleep and may feel tired and exhausted the next day. This sleep disturbance can be caused by a variety of factors, including pain, anxiety or nightmares. To help children who frequently wake up at night, parents can try to improve the child's sleep environment by providing a calm and relaxing atmosphere and keeping the bedroom dark and cool. Another sleep disorder that can occur in children is sleepwalking. Children who suffer from sleepwalking may get up and walk around at night without realizing what they are doing. This sleep disorder can be frightening for parents, but it is usually harmless and occurs in most children between the ages of 4 and 8. If a child is sleepwalking frequently, it is important to make the bedroom safe to minimize the risk of injury. Parents should also try to gently guide the child back to bed when they are sleepwalking. Another common sleep disorder in children is snoring. Although snoring can be normal in children, it can also be a sign of an underlying sleep disorder, such as obstructive sleep apnea. Children with obstructive sleep apnea have difficulty breathing regularly and may have pauses in breathing during sleep, leading to fatigue and difficulty concentrating the next day.

Sleep disorders in teenagers

Sleep disorders in teenagers are a common problem that can have a variety of causes. In fact, many teenagers suffer from sleep problems that can range from occasional sleep deprivation to serious sleep disorders. In this article, we will look at the causes, symptoms and possible treatments for sleep disorders in teenagers. Causes of teenage sleep disorders There are many possible causes of teenage sleep disorders. Here are some of the most common: Biological factors: Puberty is a time of major changes in the body, including hormonal fluctuations that can affect sleep patterns. Some studies show that teenagers' need for sleep can be up to two hours later than that of adults due to these biological factors. Technology: The constant use of cell phones, computers and other electronic devices can affect sleep quality. The blue light emitted from these devices can disrupt the production of the sleep hormone melatonin, which can lead to insomnia. Stress: Teenagers can be stressed by school pressure, social problems or family conflicts, which can lead to sleep disorders. One study has shown that stress-related sleep disorders are more common in adolescents during puberty than in children or adults. Lifestyle: An unhealthy lifestyle, including poor diet and lack of physical activity, can also cause sleep disorders in teenagers. Symptoms of teen sleep disorders Symptoms of teen sleep disorders can vary from person to person, but here are some of the most common symptoms: Trouble falling asleep: Teens with sleep disorders may have difficulty falling asleep or take a long time to fall asleep. Frequent waking: Teens may also have difficulty sleeping through the night or wake up frequently and have trouble falling back asleep. Daytime sleepiness: teens with sleep disorders may be tired or sleepy during the day and have difficulty concentrating on their activities. Mood changes: Sleep disorders can also lead to mood changes, such as irritability, anxiety and depression. Treating teen sleep disorders

When a teen suffers from sleep disorders, it's important to get a professional diagnosis and appropriate treatment. Here are some of the possible treatment options: Lifestyle changes: making healthy lifestyle changes can help reduce teen sleep disorders.

Sleep disorders in adults

Sleep disorders in adults are a common problem that affects many people. These disorders can take various forms and can have an impact on physical and mental health. In this article, we will take a closer look at sleep disorders in adults and explore the different types of sleep disorders, their causes and possible treatments. Sleep disorders can be divided into several categories, including falling asleep and staying asleep, restless sleep, excessive daytime sleepiness, sleep-related breathing disorders and parasomnias (behavioral and movement disorders during sleep). Difficulty falling asleep and staying asleep are common problems and affect many people, especially older adults. The causes of sleep disorders can vary and can range from medical problems such as sleep apnea, restless legs syndrome and pain to psychological problems such as anxiety and depression. Some sleep disorders can also occur due to lifestyle factors such as irregular sleeping habits, excessive caffeine consumption and poor diet. Insomnia and sleep disorders can be treated in various ways. One option is to change sleeping habits. This includes creating a relaxing sleep environment, maintaining a regular sleep schedule and avoiding stimulants such as caffeine and alcohol. Another option is to take medication such as sleeping pills, although these can have long-term negative effects and should therefore only be used in the short term. For sleep-related breathing disorders such as sleep apnea, continuous positive airway pressure (CPAP) therapy can be used to keep the airway open. Losing weight and avoiding alcohol and smoking can also be helpful. For restless legs syndrome, there are various medications that can be used to relieve symptoms. If sleep disorders are due to psychological issues, psychotherapeutic approaches such as Cognitive Behavioral Therapy (CBT) can be helpful. These approaches focus on identifying and addressing emotional and cognitive factors that may be contributing to the sleep disorder. In some cases, a combination of different treatment approaches may be required to effectively treat sleep disorders. It is also important to note that it may take time and patience to find an effective treatment. It may also be helpful to work with a doctor or therapist to determine the best course of action.

Sleep disorders in the elderly

Sleep disorders in the elderly are a common problem that can impact their health and quality of life. In the following, I will discuss the causes of sleep disorders in older people and some measures that can help to treat or prevent these disorders. It is generally known that older people suffer from sleep disorders more often than younger people. The reasons for this are varied and can be both physical and psychological. For example, physical illnesses such as pain, breathing problems or bladder problems can make it difficult to fall asleep or sleep through the night. Mental illnesses such as depression or anxiety disorders can also have a negative impact on sleep. Another factor that can contribute to sleep disorders in older people is the body's natural ageing process. Older people produce less melatonin, a hormone that is responsible for regulating the sleep-wake cycle. Older people can also lose muscle mass, which can lead to poorer regulation of body temperature. This in turn can lead to older people freezing or sweating more quickly at night and therefore sleeping less well. Another factor that can contribute to sleep disorders in older people is the use of medication. Many older people regularly take medication that can have a negative effect on their sleep. For example, some blood pressure medications or antidepressants can impair sleep. There are various measures that can be taken to treat or prevent sleep disorders in older people. For example, it can be helpful to pay attention to a healthy lifestyle. This includes a balanced diet, regular exercise and avoiding excessive alcohol and nicotine consumption. Good sleep hygiene can also help to prevent sleep disorders in older people. This includes, for example, keeping the bedroom as dark, quiet and cool as possible. A regular bedtime and a fixed routine before going to bed can also help older people to fall asleep more quickly and sleep better through the night. If physical or mental illnesses are the cause of sleep disorders, medical treatment may be necessary. For example, pain medication or medication for depression can be prescribed to alleviate symptoms and improve sleep. There are also alternative treatment methods that can help with sleep disorders. For example, behavioral therapy can help older people learn to deal with anxiety and worry.

Insomnia

Insomnia is a common sleep disorder that affects a person's ability to fall asleep or stay asleep. It can also cause a person to feel tired or exhausted during the day. Insomnia can be occasional or long-term and can occur in both adults and children. A person with insomnia has difficulty falling asleep or staying asleep despite spending enough time in bed. It can also affect the quality of sleep, meaning that despite getting enough sleep time, a person is still tired or exhausted in the morning. Insomnia can also cause a person to wake up early and not be able to fall back asleep. There are different types of insomnia, including primary and secondary insomnia. Primary insomnia occurs without an identifiable cause and can occur due to psychological, physiological or behavioral factors. Secondary insomnia, on the other hand, occurs due to another underlying illness or medical condition, such as pain, depression or anxiety. The symptoms of insomnia can vary from person to person. Some people have difficulty falling asleep, while others have difficulty sleeping through the night or wake up early. Other symptoms may include fatigue, sleepiness during the day, irritability, concentration problems and memory problems. There are several factors that can increase a person's risk of insomnia. These include stress, anxiety, depression, pain, irregular sleeping habits, caffeinated drinks or alcohol consumption and certain medications. There are several ways to treat insomnia. Some people can improve their sleep problems by making lifestyle changes, such as sticking to a set sleep schedule, avoiding caffeine in the late afternoon or evening and avoiding alcohol before bedtime. Others may benefit from using relaxation techniques or cognitive behavioral therapy. In some cases, a doctor may also prescribe medication to help treat insomnia. These medications can help improve sleep quality and increase sleep time. However, it is important to be aware that these medications can have side effects and that they are not suitable for everyone. There are also alternative therapies that can help treat insomnia, such as acupuncture, massage or herbal supplements. However, it is important to be aware that there is limited scientific evidence to prove the effectiveness of these therapies.

Narcolepsy

Narcolepsy is a rare neurological disorder characterized by sudden bouts of sleep during the day. The symptoms of narcolepsy can also include sleep paralysis, hallucinations and disturbed sleep at night. Narcolepsy can significantly affect the affected person's quality of life, as they may have difficulty staying awake at work or in social situations. Causes of narcolepsy The exact causes of narcolepsy are unknown, but it is thought to be an autoimmune disorder in which the immune system attacks the neurons in the hypothalamus, a part of the brain responsible for regulating the sleep-wake cycle. There is also a genetic component to narcolepsy, as the condition tends to run in some families. Symptoms of narcolepsy The main symptoms of narcolepsy are uncontrollable sleep attacks during the day. These can occur at any time, regardless of activity or caffeine intake. A typical sleep attack lasts between 10 and 20 minutes, but sometimes they can last longer. Some people with narcolepsy also have sleep paralysis, where they are unable to move while waking or falling asleep. Others have hallucinations that are often associated with falling asleep or waking up. Narcolepsy can also affect sleep at night. People with narcolepsy may have unusual sleep patterns at night, such as frequent awakenings or falling asleep quickly. Disturbed night-time sleep can lead to daytime sleepiness and drowsiness, which can exacerbate the sleep attacks. Diagnosis of narcolepsy The diagnosis of narcolepsy can be difficult, as the symptoms can also occur in other disorders. However, there are specific tests that can be performed by a sleep physician to diagnose narcolepsy. One such test is the Multiple Sleep Latency Test (MSLT), in which the patient takes several naps during the day and the time it takes to fall asleep is measured. If the patient falls asleep within five minutes, this is considered an indication of narcolepsy. Treatment of narcolepsy There is no cure for narcolepsy, but there are treatments that can alleviate the symptoms. One of the main treatments for narcolepsy is the use of stimulants such as modafinil or methylphenidate, which can help to reduce sleepiness and increase alertness.

Sleep apnea

Sleep apnea is a common sleep disorder in which sleep is interrupted by short, recurring pauses in breathing. These breathing interruptions can occur several times an hour and can result in the body not getting enough oxygen, which can lead to health problems. The symptoms of sleep apnea can vary greatly and range from loud snoring noises to tiredness and irritability during the day. In this article, we will take a closer look at sleep apnoea and its causes, symptoms and treatment options. Causes The causes of sleep apnea are not fully understood, but it is thought to be caused by a combination of genetic and environmental factors. There are certain factors that can increase a person's risk of sleep apnea, such as obesity, age, male gender, smoking and alcohol consumption. There are also certain medical conditions that can increase a person's risk of sleep apnea, such as diabetes, high blood pressure and heart disease. Symptoms The symptoms of sleep apnea can vary greatly and depend on the severity of the condition. The most common symptoms include loud snoring, pauses in breathing during sleep, sudden awakening with shortness of breath, daytime tiredness, difficulty concentrating, irritability and depression. In severe sleep apnoea, the symptoms can be more serious and lead to cardiovascular diseases such as high blood pressure, heart attacks and strokes. Diagnosis Sleep apnea is usually diagnosed by an overnight stay in a sleep laboratory or by using a portable device to monitor sleep at home. During the test, various body responses such as breathing patterns, blood oxygen levels, heart rate and brain activity are measured to determine whether sleep apnea is present and how severe it is. Treatment There are various treatment options for sleep apnea, depending on the severity and individual situation of the patient. One option is continuous positive airway pressure (CPAP) therapy, which uses a mask-like device during sleep to maintain air pressure to prevent breathing cessations. Other treatment options include lifestyle changes such as weight loss, avoiding alcohol and smoking, and the use of mouthpieces or surgery.

Restless legs syndrome

Restless legs syndrome (RLS) is a disorder of the nervous system characterized by uncomfortable sensations in the legs, particularly in the calves. The condition usually occurs at rest and disappears with movement. However, it can also disrupt sleep, which can lead to sleep disturbances and daytime sleepiness. The cause of RLS is not yet fully understood, but it is thought that both genetic and environmental factors may play a role. One of the theories is that RLS is due to a dopamine imbalance in the brain. Dopamine is a neurotransmitter that is responsible for controlling movement, mood and motivation in the brain. The symptoms of RLS can vary from person to person, but the most common are tingling, pulling, stinging or pain in the legs, usually starting in the evening or at night. The symptoms can also spread to other parts of the body such as the arms, hands or feet. The sensation is so uncomfortable that it forces the sufferer to move or massage their legs to get relief. RLS can also have an impact on sleep. The discomfort can prevent the sufferer from falling asleep or they may wake up in their sleep. People with RLS tend to have restless sleep, which can lead to tiredness and fatigue the next day. To diagnose RLS, physical examinations and blood tests are usually carried out to rule out other possible causes of the symptoms. A sleep study can also be carried out to investigate the effects of RLS on sleep. There are several treatment options for RLS, including medication, lifestyle changes and alternative therapies. Medications prescribed for RLS include dopamine agonists, benzodiazepines and anticonvulsants. Lifestyle changes such as regular exercise and stretching and avoiding alcohol and caffeine can also help to relieve the symptoms of RLS. Alternative therapies such as acupuncture and massage can also provide relief. People with RLS should also maintain healthy sleep hygiene to minimize their symptoms. This includes maintaining a regular sleep schedule, avoiding electronic devices in the bedroom and creating a relaxed sleeping environment. RLS can have a significant impact on quality of life. People with RLS can feel limited by their symptoms and it can also have an impact on their interpersonal relationships.

Periodic limb movements during sleep

Periodic limb movements during sleep (PLMS for short) are involuntary muscle movements that occur during sleep. These movements typically occur in the legs, but can also occur in the arms or other parts of the body. They can disrupt sleep and lead to tiredness and fatigue during the day. PLMS is often associated with restless legs syndrome (RLS), as both conditions are associated with restless legs and sleep disturbances. However, RLS is a separate disorder and not all people with PLMS also have RLS. In fact, some people may have PLMS without even realizing it. The exact causes of PLMS are not yet fully understood. However, there are some factors that can increase the risk of PLMS, such as certain medications, iron deficiency and neurological diseases such as Parkinson's or multiple sclerosis. There is also a genetic component, as PLMS tends to run in families. PLMS usually occurs during non-REM sleep, especially in the early stages of sleep. The movements are often rhythmic and repeat every 20-40 seconds. Although most people with PLMS do not experience pain during sleep, the movements can disrupt sleep and lead to daytime sleepiness. PLMS can occur in people of any age, but is more common in older adults. It also affects men more often than women. PLMS can be diagnosed through a physical examination and a review of sleep patterns. A doctor may also order a polysomnography to monitor the activity of the muscles during sleep. There are several treatment options for PLMS. In some cases, treating the underlying condition, such as iron deficiency, may be enough to relieve PLMS symptoms. There are also medications such as dopamine agonists and benzodiazepines that can be used to treat PLMS. However, it is important to talk to a doctor to choose the right treatment option, as some medications can have side effects. There are also some behaviors that can help reduce the symptoms of PLMS. Avoiding stimulants such as caffeine and nicotine can help improve sleep. Regular physical activity and stretching can also help to reduce symptoms. It is also important to maintain a regular sleep schedule and create a relaxing sleep environment to promote sleep. While PLMS can be bothersome, it is not usually a serious condition. However, it can lead to sleep disturbances and daytime sleepiness, which has a negative impact on quality of life. Parasomnias Parasomnias are unusual behaviors, sensations or experiences that occur during sleep and can disrupt sleep patterns. These are disturbances that can occur between waking up and falling asleep, but also during sleep itself. They can impair the experience of dreams or lead to inexplicable movements and actions. Parasomnias can occur in children and adults, and they can come in different forms. There are different types of parasomnias, each with different symptoms. Some of the most common types of parasomnias are: Sleepwalking: This is a parasomnia that can occur in children and adults. Sleepwalkers usually walk in their sleep and cannot remember anything when they wake up. Sleepwalking can be dangerous as people who sleepwalk are prone to accidents.

Nightmares

Nightmares are unpleasant dreams that are usually associated with fear or panic. They can occur in children and adults and can be caused by various factors, such as stress or anxiety. Sleep paralysis: This is a parasomnia where you feel trapped in your sleep and are unable to move or speak. Sleep paralysis can be very frightening, but it is usually harmless. Teeth grinding: Teeth grinding is a parasomnia where you grind your teeth in your sleep. This can lead to dental problems and temporomandibular joint disorders. Restless leg syndrome: Restless leg syndrome is a parasomnia characterized by unpleasant sensations in the legs that can lead to involuntary movements. This can disrupt sleep and lead to fatigue during the day. Sleep apnea Sleep apnea is a disorder in which breathing is briefly interrupted during sleep. This can lead to tiredness and other health problems. The causes of parasomnias are varied and can range from a genetic predisposition to certain medications. Other factors such as stress, lack of sleep or sleep disorders can also play a role. The treatment of parasomnias depends on the type of disorder. Some parasomnias can be treated with behavioral changes such as regular sleep hygiene or relaxation exercises. Other disorders may require medication or behavior modification therapy. It is also important to determine if there is an underlying medical condition such as depression or anxiety. Sleepwalking, also known as somnambulism, is a sleep disorder in which a person gets up and walks around in their sleep without being aware of what they are doing. The person may be very clumsy and disoriented during this stage and may even speak or interact without remembering it later. Sleepwalking is a relatively rare phenomenon, affecting around 1-15% of the population. It usually occurs in children and disappears during adulthood. However, in some people it can persist into adulthood. The exact causes of sleepwalking are unknown, but it is thought to be caused by a combination of factors such as genetic predispositions, lack of sleep, stress or anxiety, sleep apnea or certain medications. It can also occur due to fever or other physical illnesses. Sleepwalking usually occurs in the first few hours of sleep while the person is in the deep sleep phase. During this phase, the brain is not as active as during the REM phase when we normally dream. Therefore, it is not uncommon for sleepwalkers to have no memory of their nocturnal activities. Symptoms of sleepwalking can vary greatly, but they usually include getting out of bed and walking or wandering around the room or house. Sometimes, affected individuals may even leave the house or engage in dangerous activities without realizing it. These activities can range from innocent activities such as eating or dressing to dangerous activities such as driving or cooking. Although sleepwalking does not usually cause serious problems, some people can be injured while sleepwalking by bumping into objects or falling. Others may get into trouble due to their actions or lack of awareness of their surroundings. Diagnosing sleepwalking can be difficult, as many people who suffer from it do not remember what they have done. In some cases, a polysomnography can be performed, which records brain waves, muscle activity, eye movements and breathing during sleep. There are various treatment options for sleepwalking. Some people find relief by changing their sleep environment or by taking sedatives. In severe cases, therapy with medication or even surgery may be recommended. There are also some steps people can take to prevent sleepwalking from occurring. These include sticking to a regular sleep schedule, avoiding stress.

Night terrors

Night terrors, also known as sleep terrors, are a type of sleep disorder that can occur in adults and children. It usually occurs during the non-REM sleep stages and is characterized by sudden episodes of extreme anxiety, fear or panic. The affected person may stand up, scream or lash out without being fully awake or remembering the experience. In this article, we will take a closer look at night terrors and their causes, symptoms and treatment options. Causes of night terrors There is no single cause of night terrors. However, some factors that can trigger night terrors are: Lack of sleep or interruptions to sleep Stress and anxiety Sleep apnea or other sleep disorders Genetic predisposition Fever or illness Alcohol or drug use Some medications such as antidepressants Symptoms of night terrors The symptoms of night terrors are often very distressing for the person affected and for those around them. Some of the most common symptoms are Screaming or shouting Sweaty palpitations or accelerated heartbeat Restless tossing and turning Startle or sudden awakening Lack of awareness or memory of the incident Confusion or disorientation Fear or panic Most episodes of night terrors last about 10-15 minutes and end on their own. The affected person then returns to a deep sleep with no memory of the incident. Treatment of night terrors Night terrors can occur in both children and adults and can have a serious impact on the affected person's quality of life. Treatment is therefore often necessary to alleviate the symptoms and improve the quality of sleep. Psychotherapy can help to reduce stress and anxiety and thus alleviate the symptoms of night terrors. Medication: In some cases, medication may be considered. Benzodiazepines or antidepressants may be prescribed to reduce symptoms. Behavioral changes: Behavioral changes such as regular sleep-wake cycles, relaxation exercises and avoiding alcohol or caffeine can help reduce night terrors. Therapy for sleep disorders: If night terrors are associated with other sleep disorders such as sleep apnea or narcolepsy, treatment for these disorders can help reduce the symptoms of night terrors. Nightmares Sleep disorders can lead to nightmares, which can impair sleep patterns and affect general well-being. Nightmares are unpleasant dreams that can trigger strong emotional reactions such as fear, panic or anger. These dreams can feel and look different for each person. Sleep disorders can be caused by various factors such as stress, anxiety, sleep apnea, depression or irregular sleeping habits. In people with sleep disorders, nightmares can occur more frequently and be more intense than in people without sleep problems. The most common nightmares in sleep disorders are nightmares of chases, accidents or violence. These dreams can be very realistic and give the feeling that they are actually happening. It can be difficult to recover from these dreams and they can haunt the person for a long time after waking up. Another common nightmare in insomnia is dreaming of loss or separation from loved ones. These dreams can be particularly emotional and leave the person feeling sad or lonely after waking up. They can also cause the person to have difficulty falling back asleep or staying asleep. Nightmares during insomnia can also trigger physical symptoms such as sweating, palpitations or shortness of breath. These symptoms can wake the person from sleep and make it difficult to fall asleep. Insomnia and nightmares can become a vicious cycle where the fear of nightmares leads to insomnia, which in turn leads to more nightmares. There are several ways to treat nightmares in sleep disorders. One way is to treat the underlying sleep disorder. This may include establishing a regular sleep schedule, learning relaxation techniques or attending therapy to manage stress or anxiety. Another treatment option is the use of medication. Antidepressants or anxiety medications can help treat nightmares and sleep disorders. However, it is important to speak to a doctor before taking any medication to ensure there are no unwanted side effects. Relaxation techniques such as yoga, meditation or progressive muscle relaxation can also help to reduce nightmares. These techniques can help to calm the body and mind and alleviate stress-related sleep disorders. Another option is cognitive behavioral therapy (CBT). CBT can help to change negative thought patterns and learn new coping strategies.

REM sleep behavior disorder

REM sleep behavior disorder, also known as RBD (Rapid Eye Movement Sleep Behavior Disorder), is a neurological disorder in which people dream uncontrollably and intensely during REM (Rapid Eye Movement) sleep and physically act out their dreams. This can lead to injury if the person hits themselves or falls while asleep. RBD is most common in older men, but can also occur in women and younger people. Symptoms The symptoms of RBD can vary, but they usually occur during REM sleep and can include: Sleepwalking Startling out of sleep with feelings of panic or fear Physical movements, such as hitting, kicking, jumping, throwing or rolling over Speaking out loud, shouting or making other noises Sweating and rapid heartbeat Injuries that occur during sleep, such as abrasions, bruises or fractures. Causes The exact cause of RBD is unknown, but it is thought to be associated with a brain malfunction related to the regulation of REM sleep. During REM sleep, the body should normally remain relaxed to prevent movements that may result from dreaming. However, in people with RBD, this relaxation does not occur, which can lead to the physical movements. Some factors that have been associated with a higher risk of developing RBD are. RBD is more common in older people Gender: Men are more commonly affected than women Neurological conditions: RBD may be associated with some neurological conditions such as Parkinson's disease and multiple sclerosis Brain injuries: RBD may also be related to brain injuries. The diagnosis of RBD usually requires a thorough evaluation of the patient's sleep history and monitoring of sleep. A polysomnography (PSG) is a sleep study used to record behavior and activities during sleep. This study can help monitor REM sleep and physical movements during sleep. Treatment for RBD can vary depending on the severity of the symptoms and the underlying causes. In some cases, it may be sufficient to make the sleeping area safer to prevent injury. This may involve using barriers or pillows to limit the space around the bed. In more severe cases, medication such as clonazepam may be prescribed to reduce the symptoms of RBD.

Sleep related movement disorders

Sleep-related movement disorders include a variety of conditions in which uncontrolled movements or activities occur during sleep. These disorders can disrupt sleep and lead to a variety of physical and psychological problems. This article explains some of the most common sleep-related movement disorders and discusses their causes, symptoms and treatment options. One of the most common sleep-related movement disorders is restless legs syndrome (RLS), also known as Willis-Ekbom disease. With RLS, sufferers experience an unpleasant tingling or pulling sensation in the legs that can only be relieved by movement. This can lead to difficulty falling asleep and disturbed sleep. The cause of RLS is unknown, but it is thought that a disorder in the brain's dopamine system plays a role. Treatment often includes medications that affect the dopamine system, as well as lifestyle changes such as improving sleep hygiene and regular physical activity. Another common sleep-related movement disorder is periodic leg movement disorder (PLMD). This involves rhythmic movements of the legs during sleep, which can disrupt sleep. Unlike RLS, however, those affected do not feel any tingling or pulling in their legs. The cause of PLMD is also unknown, but it is thought to be linked to the dopamine system. Treatment for PLMD can be similar to RLS, including medication, sleep hygiene and regular physical activity. Another movement disorder that can disrupt sleep is REM sleep behavior disorder (RBD). In RBD, uncontrolled movements occur during REM sleep, often accompanied by vivid dreams. This can lead to injury as sufferers often perform physical activities associated with dreaming. RBD is more common in older people and can be associated with neurodegenerative diseases such as Parkinson's disease. Treatment for RBD may include medication and lifestyle changes, such as avoiding stimulants and improving sleep hygiene. Sleepwalking is another movement disorder that can disrupt sleep. It involves repeatedly getting up and walking during sleep. Sleepwalkers are often disoriented and cannot remember their activities when they wake up. Sleepwalking is more common in children, but can also occur in adults.

Bruxism

Bruxism is a condition in which a person unconsciously clenches or grinds their teeth, especially at night during sleep. It is a relatively common phenomenon that occurs in many people, especially those who suffer from stress or anxiety. However, bruxism can also occur for other reasons, such as medication, alcohol consumption or dental problems. The symptoms of bruxism can vary from person to person. Some people may show no symptoms, while others may experience severe pain or discomfort due to bruxism. The most common symptoms of bruxism include toothache, sensitive teeth, jaw pain, headaches and earaches. The exact causes of bruxism are not fully understood, but there are several factors that can contribute to the development of this condition. Stress and anxiety are common triggers of bruxism as they can lead to increased muscle tone. This can cause the person to clench or grind their teeth without realizing it. Dental problems such as tooth decay, tooth loss or an uneven bite can also trigger bruxism. Another cause of bruxism can be a certain medication or substance. Antidepressants, antipsychotics and certain allergy medications can all trigger bruxism. Alcohol consumption can also be a trigger for bruxism, as alcohol can affect muscle tone in the jaw area. Diagnosing bruxism can be difficult as many people don't even realize they have the condition. However, a thorough examination by a dentist or orthodontist can help diagnose bruxism. The dentist or orthodontist will examine the teeth, jaw and muscles around the mouth to determine if signs of bruxism are present. The treatment of bruxism depends on the severity of the condition and the underlying causes. In mild cases of bruxism, no treatment may be required as the condition does not cause severe symptoms. In more severe cases, various treatment options can be used. One option is to use a splint or mouth guard to protect the teeth during sleep and reduce pressure on the jaw. Another option is the use of muscle relaxers, which can reduce the muscle tone in the jaw area. In some cases, psychotherapy may also be required to treat stress and anxiety.

Hypersomnia

Hypersomnia is a sleep disorder in which those affected regularly suffer from excessive sleepiness and an increased need for sleep. Unlike narcolepsy, where sleep attacks and sudden loss of muscle control can occur, hypersomnia is a sleep disorder where sufferers are unable to feel rested and refreshed, even after a sufficient amount of sleep. People with hypersomnia may have difficulty staying awake, even during important or interesting activities. They may also have difficulty concentrating or completing tasks as they constantly have to fight their sleepiness. Hypersomnia can also increase the risk of accidents and injuries as sufferers can fall asleep more easily during the day. The causes of hypersomnia are not fully understood, but there are some factors that may contribute. Genetic factors may play a role, as it is more common in people whose family members are also affected. Another possible cause is a disorder in the brain that disrupts the normal sleep-wake cycle, or a dysfunction in the production or uptake of neurotransmitters such as dopamine or serotonin. Hypersomnia can also occur as a side effect of other illnesses such as depression, anxiety disorders or sleep apnea. Medications such as antidepressants or antihistamines can also cause hypersomnia. The diagnosis of hypersomnia requires a comprehensive examination to rule out other sleep disorders and make an accurate diagnosis. The examination usually includes a thorough medical history, a physical examination and tests to assess the sleep-wake cycle. These may include polysomnography (PSG), multiple sleep latency tests (MSLT) and actigraphy tests to assess the patient's sleep patterns and needs. The treatment of hypersomnia depends on the cause. For some patients, simple lifestyle changes such as regular exercise, a balanced diet and avoidance of stimulants such as caffeine and nicotine may be sufficient to relieve symptoms. For other patients, drug therapy may be necessary to reduce the need for sleep and increase alertness during the day. Stimulants such as methylphenidate and amphetamines may be prescribed to increase wakefulness, while modafinil and armodafinil may help to normalize sleep patterns.

Idiopathic hypersomnia

Idiopathic hypersomnia (IH) is a rare sleep disorder characterized by excessive daytime sleepiness and unusually long sleep times. This disorder is referred to as idiopathic because its cause is unknown and there are no known underlying medical or neurological conditions that can cause it. The symptoms of IH can be very disruptive and severely impact the daily life of the affected person. The most common symptoms include recurrent episodes of excessive sleepiness during the day, regardless of the amount and quality of sleep at night. Sufferers often complain of still feeling tired despite long periods of sleep. A person with IH may have difficulty concentrating during the day and completing tasks that require attention, which can lead to impairment at school or work. Although IH is a rare disorder, it can cause a significant impact on quality of life and lead to difficulty performing daily activities. It can also lead to social isolation and stigmatization as the symptoms are often misunderstood as laziness or lack of motivation. Diagnosing IH can be difficult as it can refer to other sleep disorders such as narcolepsy or sleep apnea syndrome, which have similar symptoms. To diagnose IH, a sleep physician usually performs a comprehensive examination, including a physical exam, blood work, and a polysomnographic exam, which records the activities of the brain, eyes, muscles, and heart during sleep. The treatment of IH is often difficult and there is no cure for the condition. Most treatment approaches focus on relieving symptoms and improving sleep quality. The use of stimulants such as methylphenidate or amphetamines can be effective in some patients to reduce sleepiness and improve alertness during the day. However, it is important that these medications are used under medical supervision as they can be associated with significant side effects. Non-drug approaches can also be useful in alleviating the symptoms of IH. A healthy lifestyle with regular exercise, a balanced diet and adequate sleep can help reduce daytime sleepiness. Relaxation and stress management techniques such as yoga or meditation can also help to improve sleep and alleviate symptoms.

Insomnia

Insomnia is a common problem that affects many people. It can manifest itself in various ways, such as difficulty falling asleep, waking up frequently during the night or feeling that sleep is not restful. In this article, we will take a closer look at insomnia, what the causes might be and how to deal with it. Insomnia can have many different causes. One of the most common causes is stress. When you're under stress, it can be difficult to relax and quiet your mind. When you try to fall asleep, thoughts and worries can prevent you from sleeping. Depression and anxiety can also lead to difficulty falling asleep or waking up more often than normal. Another factor that can lead to insomnia is the use of electronic devices, such as smartphones, tablets or computers, before bedtime. The blue light emitted by these devices can affect the body's sleep-wake cycle and cause you to fall asleep later than usual. Certain medications can also cause you to have difficulty falling asleep or wake up more often than usual. These include, for example, antidepressants, beta blockers and painkillers. If you suffer from insomnia, this can have an impact on your general well-being. You feel tired and exhausted during the day, which can affect your concentration and productivity. Mood can also deteriorate and irritability and nervousness can occur. There are various ways to deal with insomnia. One option is to adjust your lifestyle. This includes, for example, regular physical activity, a healthy diet and a fixed sleep routine. Relaxation exercises such as yoga or meditation can also help to calm the mind and promote sleep. Another approach to treating insomnia is the use of sleeping pills. However, these should only be taken in consultation with a doctor, as they can have side effects and can be addictive. There are also herbal supplements such as valerian or melatonin that can help to promote sleep. Another option for treating insomnia is behavioral therapy. This involves learning to identify and change the thoughts and behaviors that contribute to insomnia. Relaxation exercises and mindfulness meditation can also be part of behavioral therapy. It is also important to optimize the sleep environment to promote restful sleep. This includes, for example, keeping the bedroom dark and quiet and using a comfortable mattress.

Treatment of sleep disorders

Sleep disorders are a common problem that affects many people. There are different types of sleep disorders, such as difficulty falling asleep and staying asleep, nightmares and insomnia. Sleep disorders can lead to impaired physical and mental health and should therefore not be underestimated. This article presents various treatment options for sleep disorders. Behavioral changes Behavioral changes are one of the first treatment options for sleep disorders. This includes, among other things, establishing a fixed sleep-wake rhythm. This means trying to go to bed and get up at the same time every day. It is also helpful to optimize the sleeping environment, for example by darkening the bedroom and choosing a comfortable mattress. You should also avoid drinking alcohol or smoking before going to bed and avoid caffeinated drinks such as coffee or energy drinks. Relaxation techniques Relaxation techniques can help to calm the mind and body so that you can fall asleep better. These include progressive muscle relaxation, yoga, meditation and autogenic training. These techniques can help to reduce stress and prepare the body for sleep. Light therapy Light therapy can help with sleep disorders by regulating the sleep-wake rhythm. Light therapy can be provided either by special lamps or by spending time in a room with daylight. Ideally, light therapy should be used in the morning to wake up the body and stabilize the sleep-wake rhythm. Sleep hygiene Good sleep hygiene is essential for healthy sleep. This includes avoiding overeating and drinking before going to bed. Avoiding electronic devices such as smartphones and laptops in bed can also help to calm the mind and promote restful sleep.

Sleeping pills

Sleeping pills should only be considered as a last resort, as they can potentially lead to long-term dependence. However, if sleep disturbances occur due to anxiety or depression, it may be necessary to use prescription medication. However, it is important to use these medications only under medical supervision. Therapy Therapy can be helpful for sleep disorders if they are due to emotional problems or trauma. Cognitive behavioral therapy can help to change the thought patterns and behaviors that lead to sleep disorders. Psychotherapy can also help to resolve emotional problems. Medication for the treatment of sleep disorders Sleep disorders can have various causes, including stress, anxiety, depression, pain and other health problems. There are several medications that are used to treat sleep disorders, including over-the-counter and prescription medications. This article will review some of the common medications used to treat sleep disorders. Benzodiazepines Benzodiazepines are a class of drugs used to treat sleep disorders. They have a calming and relaxing effect and can help to improve sleep. Some common benzodiazepines used to treat sleep disorders are temazepam, lorazepam and diazepam. However, these drugs can be addictive and should only be used under medical supervision. Z-drugs Z-drugs are another class of drugs used to treat sleep disorders. They work in a similar way to benzodiazepines, but are not addictive. Some common Z-drugs are zopiclone, zolpidem and zaleplon. However, these drugs should also only be used under medical supervision. Antidepressants Some antidepressants can be used to treat sleep disorders. These medications can help to improve mood and promote sleep. Some common antidepressants used to treat sleep disorders are amitriptyline, mirtazapine and trazodone. However, these medications should only be used under medical supervision. Melatonin Melatonin is a hormone that is naturally produced in the body and regulates the sleep-wake cycle. Some people take melatonin as a dietary supplement to treat sleep disorders. Melatonin can help to improve sleep, especially in people whose sleep-wake cycle is disturbed. However, it should only be taken in the recommended dosage and should not be taken by pregnant or breastfeeding women. Antihistamines Some antihistamines, such as diphenhydramine and doxylamine, can be used to treat sleep disorders. These medications have sedative effects and can help to improve sleep. However, they should not be taken regularly and can cause drowsiness the next day in some people. Hypnotics

Hypnotics are medications specifically designed to treat sleep disorders. Some common hypnotics include eszopiclone, zolpidem and triazolam. These drugs can help to improve sleep, but should only be taken under medical supervision and for short periods of time.

Therapies for the treatment of sleep disorders

Sleep disorders are a common problem that affects many people. There are different types of sleep disorders, which have different causes and therefore require different therapeutic approaches. This article presents various therapies for the treatment of sleep disorders. Behavioral and lifestyle therapies One of the first steps in the treatment of sleep disorders is a review of the patient's behavior and lifestyle. Various therapies can be used here, including Sleep hygiene: this involves creating an optimal environment for sleep, including the use of comfortable mattresses and pillows, as well as implementing rules to promote sleep, such as avoiding stimulants before bedtime. Relaxation techniques: Relaxation techniques such as yoga, meditation and progressive muscle relaxation can help reduce stress and anxiety, which are common causes of sleep disorders. Stimulus control: This therapy involves linking sleep and bed so that the bed is only associated with sleep. If the patient lies awake in bed for more than 15 minutes, it is recommended that they get out of bed and do another activity until they are tired again. Chronotherapy: This therapy involves changing the sleep-wake rhythm. For example, the bedtime is shifted back a few hours in order to change the sleep rhythm. Cognitive behavioral therapy Cognitive behavioral therapy is a therapy that focuses on changing negative thoughts and behavioral patterns. This therapy can be helpful for sleep disorders, as many patients have negative thoughts and emotions related to sleep. In cognitive behavioral therapy, various techniques are used to identify and change negative thoughts. These include cognitive restructuring, which involves replacing negative thoughts with positive ones, and problem solving, which involves identifying the stressors that lead to sleep disorders and developing appropriate solutions.

Sleep medication

Sleep medication is often used to treat sleep disorders. These are drugs such as benzodiazepines or Z-drugs, which inhibit the activity of the central nervous system and thus promote relaxation. However, sleep medication should only be taken under medical supervision as it can lead to dependency. They should also only be used temporarily, as they do not solve the problem in the long term and can increase the risk of side effects. Behavioral changes to improve sleep A good night's sleep is important for our overall wellbeing and health. Unfortunately, many people struggle to get enough sleep or don't sleep well. However, there are a variety of behavioral changes that can be made to improve the quality and duration of sleep. Some of these behavioral changes are explained below. Create a sleep environment that is conducive to sleep. This can be achieved by reducing noise and light, regulating temperature and using comfortable bedding. A quiet, dark and cool room can help to improve sleep. Avoid caffeine, alcohol and nicotine before going to bed. These substances can disrupt sleep and lead to insomnia. It's also important to make sure you don't drink too much, as this can cause you to wake up frequently during the night to go to the toilet. Maintain a regular sleep rhythm. Go to bed at the same time every night and get up at the same time every morning, even at weekends. This helps to regulate the body's natural sleep rhythm and can help you fall asleep faster and sleep better. Avoid engaging in intense physical activity before bedtime. Exercise can keep the body and brain active and make it harder to fall asleep. However, it is important to incorporate regular physical activity into your daily routine as it can help improve the quality and duration of sleep. Avoid eating large meals before bedtime. Heavy meals can cause the body to stay active and make it harder to fall asleep. It is better to have light snacks that do not interfere with sleep. Switch off electronic devices before going to bed. The light from TVs, computers and smartphones can cause the brain to stay active and make it harder to fall asleep. It is better to avoid electronic devices for an hour before bedtime and instead do a relaxing activity such as reading or meditating. Develop a relaxation routine before bedtime. This can be achieved through activities such as reading, yoga or meditation. A relaxation routine helps the body and mind prepare for sleep and can help improve sleep. Avoid working in bed or doing other activities that are not related to sleep. The body should associate the bed with sleep and relaxation

Alternative therapies for the treatment of sleep disorders

Sleep disorders can greatly affect a person's daily life. Alternative therapies can be an effective way to treat sleep disorders, helping to regulate the sleep cycle and promote a good night's rest. Below we will describe some of the most effective alternative therapies for treating sleep disorders. Acupuncture is a traditional Chinese therapy in which thin needles are inserted into specific points on the skin to regulate the flow of vital energy in the body. This therapy can help to regulate the sleep cycle and relax the body, which can lead to better sleep. Aromatherapy involves the use of essential oils to create a calming and relaxing atmosphere. Lavender oil is one of the most popular options as it has a calming effect and prepares the body for sleep. Melatonin: Melatonin is a naturally occurring hormone produced by the body to regulate the sleep-wake cycle. It can also be taken as a dietary supplement to increase melatonin levels in the body and improve sleep. Yoga is one of the best alternative therapies for relaxation and sleep cycle regulation. It involves gentle stretching exercises and breathing techniques that can help to calm the body and mind and promote sleep. Progressive muscle relaxation involves the contraction and relaxation of specific muscle groups in the body to achieve deep relaxation. This therapy can help to reduce stress and prepare the body for sleep. Meditation: Meditation can help calm the mind and reduce stress, which can lead to improved sleep quality. There are different types of meditation, such as mindfulness meditation, transcendental meditation and yoga meditation, all of which can help improve sleep. Hypnosis: Hypnosis can be an effective alternative therapy for treating sleep disorders. It can help calm the mind and relax the body to promote deeper sleep. Music therapy: Music can have a calming and relaxing effect and help to regulate the sleep cycle. There are specific pieces of music that are recommended for the treatment of sleep disorders. Herbal medicine: Herbal medicine can also be an effective alternative therapy for treating sleep disorders.

Tips for improving sleep

Good sleep is crucial for our physical and mental health. When we get sufficient and quality sleep, we are more productive, more focused and have a better mood. Conversely, sleep problems can lead to fatigue, irritability, poor performance and poor health. In this article, I will provide tips for improving sleep. Establish a routine: Try to go to bed and get up at the same time every day, even on weekends. A routine will help your body to develop and maintain a regular sleep rhythm. Create a comfortable sleeping environment: Make sure your bedroom is cool, dark and quiet. Use comfortable bedding and pillows and make sure the mattress is comfortable. Avoid excessive caffeine consumption: Caffeine can affect sleep quality, especially if consumed in the afternoon or evening. Try to reduce or avoid caffeine consumption. Avoid alcohol and smoking: Alcohol and smoking can also affect sleep quality. Alcohol can lead to a shallow sleep phase, while nicotine is a stimulant that makes it harder to fall asleep. Avoid heavy meals before bedtime: A heavy meal can put a strain on the digestive tract and make it harder to fall asleep. Try to avoid eating large meals at least two hours before bedtime. Exercise regularly: Regular exercise can help to regulate your sleep rhythm and prepare your body for sleep. However, make sure that you don't do any intensive exercise at least three hours before going to bed, as this can affect the quality of your sleep. Relax before going to bed: Try to establish a relaxation routine before you go to bed. This can include taking a warm bath, practicing yoga, meditating or reading a book. Avoid using electronic devices before bedtime: The light from cell phones, tablets and laptops can stimulate the brain and disrupt sleep patterns. Try to avoid electronic devices for at least an hour before bedtime. Use a sleep diary: Recording sleep patterns and habits can help to identify patterns and solve problems. Note your bedtimes and how long you sleep to determine if there are patterns that need to change.

Conclusion: How to avoid sleep disorders

Sleep is an important function of our body that helps us to recover and prepare our body and mind for the next day. If we don't get enough sleep, we can feel sluggish, unfocused and irritable. In the long term, sleep disorders can lead to health problems such as heart disease, diabetes and depression. That's why it's important that we make an effort to get enough sleep and avoid sleep disorders. In this conclusion, we will summarize some tips that can help us avoid sleep disorders. One of the most important factors for good sleep is a regular routine. It is important to go to bed and get up at the same time every day to get our body used to a natural rhythm. We should also use our bedtime to relax. It is advisable to avoid activities that excite or stress us, such as work or electronic devices, about an hour before bedtime. Another important recommendation for improving sleep is to create a comfortable sleeping environment. The choice of mattress, pillow and comforter plays an important role here. The room should also be cool, dark and quiet to create an optimal sleeping environment. It is also important that we take care of our physical health to promote good sleep. We should try to be physically active and exercise, as this exhausts the body and promotes sleep. We should also try to eat healthily and avoid alcohol and caffeine, as these substances can affect our sleep. Another important factor for good sleep is stress management. Stress can keep us awake and prevent us from resting. To reduce stress, we can use techniques such as yoga, meditation or relaxation exercises. We should also try to calm our minds before going to bed, for example by reading a book or listening to music. Finally, it is important that we take care of our mental well-being to promote good sleep. Mental health issues such as anxiety or depression can prevent us from sleeping well. It is important that we take care of our mental health by seeking professional help or using self-help techniques if necessary. Overall, there are many tips and techniques that can help us avoid sleep disorders. A regular routine, a comfortable sleep environment, physical activity, healthy eating, stress management and mental wellbeing are all important factors that can help promote a good night's sleep. It is important that we make an effort to incorporate these tips into our daily lives.

Imprint

Marie Moreno
Am Anger 3
06869 Coswig
Germany
Luna-Publishing.de